Community Support for New Families

A Guide to Organizing a Postpartum Parent Support Network in Your Community

Jane I. Honikman, M.S.

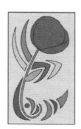

Praeclarus Press. LLC

www.praeclaruspress.com

Praeclarus Press, LLC
2504 Sweetgum Lane
Amarillo, Texas 79124 USA
806-367-9950
www.PraeclarusPress.com

DISCLAIMER

The information contained in this publication is advisory only and is not intended to replace sound clinical judgment or individualized patient care. The author disclaims all warranties, whether expressed or implied, including any warranty as the quality, accuracy, safety, or suitability of this information for any particular purpose.

ISBN: 978-0-9854180-8-3

ISBN (e-book): 978-0-9854180-9-0

Cover Design and Illustration: Ken Tackett

Developmental Editing: Kathleen Kendall-Tackett

Copy Editing: Diana Cassar-Uhl

Layout & Design: Todd Rollison

Operations: Scott Sherwood

Never doubt that a small group of thoughtful, committed citizens can change the world; indeed, it's the only thing that ever does.

- Margaret Mead (1901-1978)

In 1990, I became a mother for the first time. I was just finishing up my Ph.D. in developmental psychology, a degree which has been (and still is) valuable in my professional life. Unfortunately, it was pretty much useless for me as a new mother. It was during that time that I became acutely aware of the staggering lack of support for new mothers in the U.S. In trying to figure out what we needed to do, I looked far and wide to find groups who were effectively meeting new mothers' needs. It was during this time that I learned of Jane Honikman's work as Founder of Postpartum Support International.

As time passed, I continued my work with new mothers. As a researcher, I began to study them and document their experiences. I wrote a book about postpartum depression and included many mothers' stories. I became a La Leche League Leader and worked directly with new mothers who had concerns about breastfeeding, and often life in general. I wrote more books about early motherhood. I got to know Jane and asked her to write a Foreword for the next two editions of *Depression in New Mothers*. Some things, like earlier recognition of postpartum depression, have really gotten better. But there is still much to do.

Over the past two decades, I've observed that when a community supports its new parents, it has substantially lower rates of breastfeeding difficulties, postpartum depression, and even child abuse. These are tremendous problems, and the long-term cost is enormous. Wouldn't it be better to prevent them in the first place? Providing effective support for new families could do just that. It's no wonder that the late Ray Helfer, M.D., pediatrician and pioneer in the child maltreatment field, called the postpartum period a "window of opportunity for intervening with new families." It's a time when families are quite vulnerable, but are most open to receiving information about how to be good parents.

So how can we work to provide this support to families in our communities? I'm glad you asked.

In this book, Jane Honikman shares her four decades of experience in creating organizations that work with new parents. It is a step-by-step guide that shows you how to start an organization that will care for new families in your communities. I've been involved with starting a couple of organizations. As I read Jane's book, I found myself thinking, "Wow, this would have been really helpful to know earlier."

Community Support for New Families is formatted like a workbook. It will walk you through the process of forming a group, and putting things in place to ensure its long-term survival. Jane addresses many of the issues that can cause a group to fail. And she encourages us to think about creating an organization that will outlast us.

In short, Jane shows us that a few determined people can indeed change the world: step by step, one family at a time. Thank you for taking the first step towards supporting new families in your community. Please know that it does make a difference.

Kathleen Kendall-Tackett
February 11, 2013
Amarillo, Texas

My goal in writing this workbook is to encourage individuals to work as a team to support parents and their families. Although the world comprises countless different cultures, in each there are parents and children. This workbook provides a guideline or framework for committed individuals to create support systems that will endure. Although it has been designed primarily for use in the United States and Canada, it can easily be adapted to work in other countries.

The definition of a parent-support network is broad. I often use the terms "group" and "network" interchangeably. A parent-support group, or network, can be an ongoing support group, a collaboration between agencies, an informational service, or a clearinghouse. All have in common a commitment to assist families by providing information and emotional support.

My experience began in the 1970s through the cofounding of Postpartum Education for Parents (PEP). In 1979, I coauthored a guidebook on how we achieved our vision. I learned that careful planning and goal setting can build a strong organization; PEP endures because we followed specific and practical steps.

In 1987, I founded Postpartum Support International (PSI) to represent self-help groups working in the prevention or alleviation of negative emotional reactions to childbearing. I had discovered that there were other groups similar to PEP. We needed to share our experiences and build a global network. Although PSI does not create or fund any support groups, the organization empowers and encourages interested individuals to create them and to strengthen existing support groups.

Establishing a support group and/or network is a very individual experience. There is no rigid and absolute recipe. This individuality allows personalization and creativity, but it can be overwhelming in the face of so many decisions. This workbook contains a practical outline of stages and steps to help you through the process. It doesn't provide a timeline, because the pacing is as individual as the organizers and their communities.

In this workbook and in your own research, you will read about a wide variety of groups and their experiences. They have different philosophies, services, and structures. What they all have in common, though, is that they comprise concerned people who have committed their time, talents, and patience to creating services to benefit other families. I mention specific groups in order to communicate that there's no single right way to develop and maintain a parent-support network. Take the initiative and use the list of organizations in Appendix B to contact some of these groups. The process of completing this workbook will help you make personal connections with others in the field. They are your resources, peers, and pioneers.

This workbook has been divided into six stages. As you read and work through them, you'll realize that many of the stages and steps can be done simultaneously. It's a good idea to read the entire workbook initially, review some of the concepts, and then work each step in order. Stages 1 and 2 are the beginning.

Stage 1 asks you to visualize and start an organization for the parent-support network you would like to create. You need to find others who share your vision and commitment to make this network real and viable.

Stage 2 requires you to research other parent-support groups and networks that already exist in your community and beyond. The information and personal connections that you start to make in this stage will shape your decisions in the subsequent stages of this workbook.

Stage 3, the Planning Stage, is the most time consuming. It involves the "meat" of this work process. Starting with Step 1, you will begin to formulate your group's purpose, philosophy, goals, and objectives, which from now on I will call the PPGO. In addition, you will make decisions regarding the services to provide and the group structure. There is a discussion of funding, along with volunteer and staff issues.

Stage 4 is about implementing the group's services. The contacts that you developed in previous stages will help you form an advisory board of professionals who serve your target population. The ideas that you and the core committee developed earlier will be turned into printed material and will represent your group. Through your group's outreach efforts, the general community starts to hear about what the new network will offer them. The last step is the implementation of service.

Stage 5 can feel both concrete and abstract. You deliver services; there's something to show for your hard work and vision. Yet it can feel anticlimactic when the participation level starts low or drops off. If your group offers emotional support, the volunteers or service deliverers may not be able to measure the effects of their interventions/services. There are methods for evaluating a group's effectiveness, but this part of the process is often neglected. Without Stage 5, your group cannot endure.

Stage 6 encourages you to develop partnerships outside your group and to have an influence on the services of other organizations in your local community. You'll learn how to set new goals and objectives to keep your group fresh and vital, and, should you care to, how to write your own account of starting the network.

I've learned from my experience over the last four decades that it's crucial to create a structure in order to produce success. If this structure is appropriate, strong, and adaptable, your group will touch the lives of many families and have a lasting influence.

I can summarize my 40 years of experience in organizing new parent support as follows:

- You can't do it alone.
- You need to know your goals before you begin.
- You need to be systematic in your approach.

My hope is that this workbook will empower a new generation of parent-support pioneers to realize their potential to improve our society by strengthening its core structure: the family.

Jane Honikman
Santa Barbara, CA
January, 2013

STAGE 1.
Brainstorming

STEP 1: Identify Personal Qualifications

STEP 2: Start a File

STEP 3: Create a Core Committee or Task Force

STEP 4: Choose Committee Members

STEP 5: Identify Your Target Audience

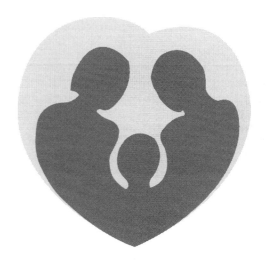

Step 1: Identify Personal Qualifications

This step will help you identify your goals and realistically assess whether you have the time and resources to accomplish them. Recognize that there could be some personal benefit in starting this organization, such as satisfaction for a job well done, recognition, or even money. There may also be personal costs. Organizations can consume a great deal of time and resources.

Goals for the Organization

In thinking about this organization, what do you hope to accomplish? What are your immediate and long-term goals for this organization?

_____
_____
_____
_____
_____
_____

Do you have the patience to see this group from conception to operation to maintenance? *Patience cannot be understated or taken lightly. It requires perseverance to work through each stage of the organizing process.*

_____
_____
_____
_____

Assessment of Your Other Obligations

What are your current life priorities and obligations?
Partner, children, employment, extended-family obligations, etc.

_____
_____
_____
_____

Do you have time to work on this project? What projects or activities will you need to put on hold while you start this group? *Recognize that the time required by the process is critical. Pledging yourself to a goal is not enough without fully acknowledging how much time it will take. Realistically estimate the amount of time it will take and double that. Will you be able to allocate that much time to this project?*

_____

_____

_____

_____

What does your spare time look like? *What days and times of the week are you available? How frequently throughout the week? Are these small pieces or long blocks of time? If you cannot work on this during the week, are you able to work evenings and weekends? Do you want to?*

_____

_____

_____

_____

Potential Benefits and Costs

What are the potential benefits of starting this organization for you and your community?

_____

_____

What are the potential costs?

_____

_____

Did a personal experience make you want to do this work? Have you sufficiently recovered from your own experience in order to assist others or work on this project?

_____

_____

_____

Have you discussed your readiness with people who know you well?

_____

_____

Do you have support in place to help you cope with any issues that may come up?

_____

_____

_____

What do you do to take care of yourself?

_____

_____

_____

Personal Skill and Knowledge Assessment

How many months do you expect to take to establish this project? Are you committed to seeing this through to the end result? *No matter who you are, a parent or a professional, the most important qualification needed to accomplish your goal is commitment.*

_____

_____

_____

If "no" but you still want to do it, what must you change in your life to become a leader?

_____

_____

If you cannot be a leader, what other role could you play?

_____

_____

_____

Do you know others who may be interested in leading?

_____

What research have you done on parent support?
Examples include word of mouth, books, training, seminars.

_____

_____

_____

What research have you done on psychological and psychiatric disorders related to pregnancy, birth, and the postpartum period?

_____

_____

_____

What research on other topics related to parenting have you done?

_____

_____

Ask yourself the following questions and complete the grid below.
- What do you know now?
- What skills do you need to acquire?
- What areas do you need to develop further during the course of your journey toward creating this organization?

Required Skill/Knowledge	Currently Have	Further Development
Leadership skills		
Listening skills		
Knowledge of normal adjustment to parenthood		
Referral knowledge		
Pregnancy and postpartum knowledge		
Knowledge of difficulties in the postpartum period		
Other: _____		

Step 2: Start a File

Once you decide to form a group, you will need to create a system that will allow you to store all your information in one place. Keep an accurate record of the information you gather. This can be done electronically or in hard copy. Start a binder or an electronic folder in which you document all your contacts and ideas. Don't forget to date your notes and list contact names, phone numbers, and e-mail addresses. There are many electronic methods for storing information in that you can share online with other people. Some of these services are free, such as Google Drive, and some are paid, such as Central Desktop or Basecamp.

YES or NO

☐ ☐   You've made a binder or filing system in which you keep relevant phone numbers and documents. You can use hard copies or an electronic shared workspace, such as Google Drive, Central Desktop, or Basecamp.

☐ ☐   This binder/filing system is easy to get to and separated from your personal, home, and work documents.

If "no," how can you prevent losing the binder and/or make it easier to get to?

_____

_____

_____

Step 3: Create a Core Committee or Task Force

Who will organize the Group or Network?

It's important to find others who share your interests in new-parent support in order to avoid burnout. These individuals you have identified are with whom you will work. You must have sympathetic people who will help with the many tasks involved in starting a new organization. You may already have people you know who would like to volunteer. Write the names and contact information for people already interested in joining this project.

Name	Phone/Email	Possible Task

Finding Others

If you are looking for others to join in your work, you can send out a "Call for Organizers." This can be distributed in electronic form via email or social media. Or you can post hard copies in places you feel are most appropriate, e.g., grocery stores, doctors' offices, libraries, community centers, and clinics. Mail copies to key people in your community. You can also have a notice published in your local newspaper or community bulletin.

Another inexpensive approach would be to write an editorial for your local paper expressing the needs of new families and a call for people who would like to do something about meeting that need. Keep these methods in mind when it comes time to recruit volunteers and members.

Identify Key Stakeholders

Who are the key people/what are the key organizations that should be involved in this effort? Check the groups/individuals that you have contacted.

YES or NO

- ☐ ☐ Your Postpartum Support International (PSI) regional coordinator
- ☐ ☐ Other self-help groups for new families
- ☐ ☐ Resource centers
- ☐ ☐ Churches/temples
- ☐ ☐ Social workers
- ☐ ☐ Schools
- ☐ ☐ Employee assistance programs
- ☐ ☐ Hospital chaplains
- ☐ ☐ Hospital social workers
- ☐ ☐ Local and state self-help clearinghouses
- ☐ ☐ Medical and mental healthcare professionals
- ☐ ☐ Family and friends
- ☐ ☐ Acquaintances and others
- ☐ ☐ Lactation consultants
- ☐ ☐ Doulas
- ☐ ☐ Childbirth educators
- ☐ ☐ Midwives
- ☐ ☐ La Leche League leaders
- ☐ ☐ Breastfeeding USA counselors
- ☐ ☐ WIC peer counselors
- ☐ ☐ Community members

Meetup

Meetup is the world's largest network of local groups. Meetup makes it easy for anyone to organize a local group or find one of the thousands already meeting up face-to-face. More than 9,000 groups get together in local communities each day, each one with the goal of improving themselves or their communities.

Meetup's mission is to revitalize local community and help people around the world self-organize. Meetup believes that people can change their personal world, or the whole world, by organizing themselves into groups that are powerful enough to make a difference.

Learn more at *meetupblog.meetup.com* .

The National Association of Mothers' Centers (NAMC)

NAMC is an example of a community organization that supports new mothers. One of the core missions of NAMC is to educate mothers and families about postpartum depression (PPD) and help them reach out for guidance and support.

As part of this effort, NAMC has collaborated with the Postpartum Resource Center of NY for the past four years to offer Circle of Caring, peer-led PPD support groups at local Mothers' Centers. The groups offer emotional support, educational information, and coping tools.

Step 4: Choose Committee Members

Providing community support for new families requires the commitment of a dedicated core of individuals. While one person may be the visionary, it is imperative that a committee or task force be formed to ensure that the group can thrive past the initial start-up phase. Your first step is to think about who you'd like to partner with you in forming the initial committee or task force.

Based on the individuals you identified in Step 3, who are possible members of your initial committee? List their names and contact information below.

Name	Phone/Email	Possible Task

YES or NO

☐ ☐ Are your committee members local?
☐ ☐ Have they agreed to meet in person on a regular basis?

Committee Meetings

What will be the dates, times, and locations of your meetings?

_____

_____

If committee members are not local, can you use online resources, such as Skype, FreeConferenceCall.com, and Google Drive?

_____

How will the committee operate? Is there a chairperson? How will that person be appointed? Who will it be?

_____

_____

Will decisions be made by consensus or majority vote?

_____

_____

Who will take the committee meeting minutes?

_____

_____

Team Cooperation

Is this committee about the needs of the organizers or those of parents in your community? Or both? *It's important that the organizers make a commitment to cooperate as a whole, and not to compete as individuals. Are there individuals on your team who might not be willing to work with others? How can you handle that situation?*

_____

_____

_____

Individual Strengths and Weaknesses

Members of the committee should recognize and take responsibility for their own strengths and weaknesses. Use the tool in Appendix A to assess this. The answers are confidential. This is just an exercise for personal growth and to help each member decide which upcoming tasks to volunteer for. Try to match tasks with team member strengths. Look at the skills and proficiencies in your task force, and work with those to develop an effective committee for your organization.

_____

_____

_____

_____

Has each organizer made a commitment to listen and show respect for other members' opinions? What are some of the differing opinions that organizers have stated so far?

_____

_____

_____

_____

> ## The National Association of Mothers' Center
>
> Since 1975, The National Association of Mothers' Centers has found it helpful to create committees from individuals who like to work in groups and who respect others through listening.

When differing opinions come up, what are some of the things that may block team cooperation?

_____

_____

_____

_____

How can the committee regain its commitment to cooperate when differing opinions arise or feelings get hurt?

_____

_____

_____

_____

How is the creation of the committee going?

_____

_____

Step 5: Identify Your Target Audience

The next step is getting more specific about who will receive your services. Below are some questions to help you think more specifically about those you want to reach.

Who will receive services provided by your organization?

YES or NO

- ☐ ☐ Pregnant women?
- ☐ ☐ Partners?
- ☐ ☐ Families struggling with adjustment to parenthood?
- ☐ ☐ Families who are stressed and distressed?
- ☐ ☐ Mothers with prenatal depression (PND) or postpartum depression (PPD)?
- ☐ ☐ Breastfeeding mothers?
- ☐ ☐ Formula-feeding parents?
- ☐ ☐ Parents of children with disabilities?
- ☐ ☐ Will mothers with miscarriage and other grief issues be invited to participate?
- ☐ ☐ May babies attend?
- ☐ ☐ May older children attend?
- ☐ ☐ May fathers attend?
- ☐ ☐ Adopting parents?
- ☐ ☐ Extended family members?
- Others?_____

Naming the Group or Organization

Names can be cute or clever, but the intent is to describe the group so potential members can easily recognize how the group will help them. "Postpartum Adjustment Group" or "Support for Mothers" are just as effective as "The Emotional You," "Beyond Baby Blues," and "Baby Makes Three." Do a Google search on the names you are considering to make sure they're not already in use. Try to incorporate as much of your goal as an organization into your title. That is how others will find you.

Proposed Group Titles

_____

_____

_____

_____

_____

Once you establish your group's name, make sure to reserve the domain name for your website (check to make sure no other group is using that name or one that is too similar to yours).

Ideas for a Logo

A logo can be useful for group name recognition, but it's not necessary. You can choose to not have one, share an existing logo, or create one yourself. Draw or describe some ideas for a logo in the space below. If there is an art school or college with an art department in your community, you might ask if any of their students would be willing to design a logo for you.

You might also check out stock photo sites, such as *Fotolia.com*. These sites have stock illustrations that can be licensed and used in a logo for very little money. A graphic designer can then add your organization's name to the stock image.

STAGE 2.
Investigation

STEP 1:   Identify Resources Already Available
           in Your Community

STEP 2:   Community Needs Assessment

STEP 3:   Interface with Other Agencies

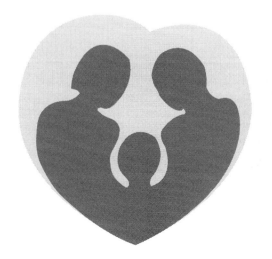

Step 1: Identify Resources Already Available in your Community

Learn what agencies/groups in your community do and who they serve. You may want to keep a separate file with their brochures or literature. Complete the table below to record your progress, and check the line at left when you are familiar with what the agency or group does. Look up websites, make calls, email listed contacts, set up meetings, and ask questions. With some groups, you may need to contact the national or international office to find out if there is a group in your community.

Have you asked the people/groups listed below for information about current resources? Check those you have contacted.

YES or NO

- ☐ ☐ Local PSI coordinator
- ☐ ☐ Social workers
- ☐ ☐ School counselors
- ☐ ☐ Therapists
- ☐ ☐ Self-help clearinghouses
- ☐ ☐ Medical and healthcare professionals
- ☐ ☐ Resource centers
- ☐ ☐ Hospital chaplains
- ☐ ☐ Human resources offices
- ☐ ☐ Hospital social workers
- ☐ ☐ Employee-assistance programs
- ☐ ☐ Attachment Parenting International
- ☐ ☐ La Leche League
- ☐ ☐ Breastfeeding USA
- ☐ ☐ Early Intervention
- ☐ ☐ Doula organizations (DONA, CAPPA)
- ☐ ☐ WIC peer counselors
- ☐ ☐ Physicians
- ☐ ☐ Child abuse prevention
- ☐ ☐ Other organizations that work with new families in your community:_____

_____

_____

_____

Record the name of the person you contacted, the organization name, and that person's contact information.

Name	Organization	Phone Number	Email

What have you learned from your contacts with existing organizations?

Postpartum Support International?

_____

Breastfeeding organizations?

_____

Parenting organizations (e.g., Attachment Parenting International)?

_____

Other agencies?

_____

What have you learned from other individuals?

Volunteers?

_____

Other parents?

_____

Step 2: Community Needs Assessment

When choosing what population you want to serve, contact people who are already working in your community. These people may be aware of needs that are not being met by existing services. Also, consider the unique characteristics of your community, or the larger group of families you want to serve.

Geographic Location

Will you be working in your own community? _____

Where is your community located? _____

Characteristics of Your Community

Ask yourself the following questions and write a brief description of your community below.

- Is your community rural or urban?
- Does it have a small or large population?
- How far is it from government services?
- How affluent is your community?
- What is the demographic and racial/ethnic distribution of your community?
- What are the primary languages spoken?
- Is there access to public transit?
- What is the education level of the families you want to reach?

_____

_____

_____

_____

If you are unsure of your community's needs, you can also develop a brief survey, and send it to key informants (including consumers) in your community. This will allow you to find out what they identify as the most pressing needs, and if those needs are already being met. It makes no sense to duplicate services that are already being offered, but you may be able to offer services that complement and extend existing services.

Calculating Anticipated Need for Your Services

Another way to assess needs in your community is to estimate the number of families who may encounter difficulties. For example, researchers have found that approximately 10% to 20% of mothers become depressed after having a baby. You can use this figure to determine the need in your community for what you want to offer, to develop fundraising literature, and to educate the public.

Community birth rate: _____
$$X\ 0.10$$
= _____ **families suffering from depression postprtum**

Breastfeeding may be another area where you can calculate the number of families that will need support. While many mothers initiate breastfeeding in the hospital, a substantial percentage will wean or supplement in the first few days and weeks. Community support is so vital to breastfeeding success that it is Step 10 of UNICEF's Baby-Friendly Hospital Initiative. The Centers for Disease Control and Prevention (CDC) offers states a Breastfeeding Report Card. This is a way to estimate the rate of breastfeeding within your state. Local hospitals may also collect this information.

What is the percentage of mothers in your state and community who initiate breastfeeding?

_____

What is the rate of exclusive breastfeeding at three months?

_____

What is the rate of exclusive breastfeeding at six months?

_____

Strengths of the Community

What services are currently available for the pregnant and postpartum population?

_____

_____

_____

Limitations of the Community

What are some of the barriers that limit families' access to services?

_____

_____

_____

What services are not available?

_____

_____

_____

Step 3: Interface with Other Agencies

Know your limitations. Make referrals.

It is unlikely that you will be able to meet all of the needs of families you serve. The good news is that you don't have to. Think of yourself as an addition or supplement to the services already offered in your community. Don't become an adversary or competitor to existing agencies. It doesn't help parents to be led to believe that only your group can give them the support they need. Unless your group can provide childcare (all the time, not just during group time), financial assistance, job training, medical advice and services, housing, marital counseling, psychiatric services, drug and alcohol services, household help, spiritual guidance, etc., your group isn't the only organization for your members. Other organizations can fill gaps in family, community, and/or professional support. There are many groups around the world whose sole functions are to provide referrals to other groups, organizations, or professionals.

By becoming aware of the services that other organizations in your area provide, you can focus your group on providing parents with what isn't already available.

Realize that your group will have a limited but important role in the lives of the parents you reach. Just as you will be able to see what other groups and organizations are missing concerning parent and perinatal support, you must be aware of your own group's limitations.

Use the list of community organizations you developed in Step 1 to identify organizations that will be part of your referral network.

Which groups might you refer families to?

_____

_____

_____

_____

_____

How will you refer consumers to these groups?

_____

_____

_____

_____

_____

_____

STAGE 3.
Planning

STEP 1:   Establish Your Purpose, Philosophy, Goals, and Objectives (PPGO)

STEP 2:   Fill in Your Actual, Agreed-Upon PPGO

STEP 3:   What Services Will Achieve Your Goals?

STEP 4:   Compare and Contrast Organizations

STEP 5:   Seek Locations

STEP 6:   Beyond the Core Committee

STEP 7:   Formalize a Budget

STEP 8:   Open a Bank Account

STEP 9:   Seek Funding

STEP 10: Recruit Volunteers and/or Hire Staff

STEP 11: Provide Training and Orientation to Volunteers and Staff

Step 1: Establish Your Purpose, Philosophy, Goals, and Objectives (PPGO)

Creating the PPGO

The purpose, or mission, is a succinct, overarching reason for the group's existence. The philosophy is a unified way of doing things. Philosophies are usually multifaceted, but you should be able to state yours concisely. Goals, or aims, like your purpose, are concrete, long-term accomplishments for your group to achieve. Objectives are specific ways to achieve your goals. Usually groups will have several goals and several objectives. While the purpose and philosophy of a group generally do not change, goals and objectives should be revised as the group evolves.

Your PPGO should be stated as clearly and accurately as possible. It provides a focus, direction, and definition for the group that the organizers and the general public will understand and be able to use. The shorter and more concise you can make your purpose, goals, and objectives, the more likely that your group will achieve them.

Proposed Purpose or Mission

Examples of Proposed Missions

Postpartum Support International's (PSI) purpose, or mission, is "to eliminate denial and ignorance of emotional health related to childbirth" and "to increase awareness among public and professional communities about the emotional changes women often experience during pregnancy and after the birth of a baby."

The mission of the National Association of Mothers' Centers (NAMC) is to create a community of women--who through mutual support and public advocacy--explore, enrich, and value the maternal experience.

La Leche League International's mission is to help mothers worldwide to breastfeed through mother-to-mother support, encouragement, information, and education and to promote a better understanding of breastfeeding as an important element in the healthy development of the baby and mother.

Proposed Philosophy

Your philosophy is your way of doing things. Implied in many existing parenting support organizations' philosophies around the world are the concepts:

1. Your postpartum experience is common/you are not alone;
2. You are not to blame for whatever you may be feeling; and
3. You will feel like yourself again.

Below are some examples.

The philosophy of Postpartum Education for Parents (PEP) in Santa Barbara, California is that "there is no one right way to parent."

The philosophy of the Pacific Postpartum Support Society (PPPSS) in Canada consists of 17 items. It includes the phrases "postpartum depression is not caused by inadequacy or failure on the part of the woman," "women are the experts on their lives," "women need a place of their own," "society offers little support for women as mothers," and "society delivers double messages about the importance of mothering."

The National Association of Mothers' Centers (NAMC) in the U.S. is a group whose philosophy is based on "maintaining a nonjudgmental attitude toward others who have ideas that are different from your own and promoting a nonhierarchical structure where each woman's voice has value." Their mission: "To enable women involved in pregnancy, adoption, and child-rearing to effectively use their individual and collective knowledge and experiences as catalysts for personal and societal changes that benefit mothers and families."

Proposed Goals or Aims

Goals and aims should be a concise sentence or two about what your organization is trying to accomplish. Some examples are listed below.

Examples of Goals and Aims

Since 1983, the Program for Early Parent Support (PEPS) organization's philosophy has been that no new parent feel isolated, ill-equipped, overwhelmed, unsupported, or insecure; that all parents develop the confidence to build strong, healthy families; and that all children grow up in a social environment that allows them to thrive.

The goals of the Program for Early Parent Support are to:

- Train volunteer leaders to foster a comfortable, informative atmosphere that encourages peer interaction and builds trust among new friends,
- Collaborate with local healthcare professionals and organizations to allow services to complement, rather than compete with, other community parenting resources, and
- Provide meetings in each other's homes to create a network of neighborhood-based support.

The goals of the National Association of Mothers' Centers are to:

- Create a network of centers, online networking, and programs by and for mothers
- Raise awareness of and promote maternal well-being
- Be a resource for its individual and center members
- Advocate for public policies that value the work of caregiving

Proposed Objectives

Objectives are concrete, time-dependent ways to achieve goals. Long-term objectives can have broad deadlines, but short-term objectives need specific deadlines. At the end of a deadline, your group needs to evaluate progress toward the objective and, if necessary, set a new deadline for it.

Example of Objectives

The short-term objectives of Postpartum Support International (PSI) are set during the Board of Trustees meetings several times during the year. These are measurable and time related.

The long-term objectives of PSI are to:

- Provide current information to members on the diagnosis and treatment of postpartum mental illness,
- Advocate for research into the etiology, diagnosis, and treatment of postpartum mental illness,
- Provide education about the mental health issues of childbearing,
- Address legal and insurance-coverage issues,
- Encourage collaboration with related organizations,
- Encourage healthcare professionals' participation in PSI,
- Encourage the formation of new groups and strengthen existing groups, and
- Sponsor an annual PSI conference to review progress in achieving these objectives.

Step 2: Fill in Your Actual Agreed-upon PPGO

Purpose

_____

_____

_____

_____

Philosophy

_____

_____

_____

_____

_____

Goals and Aims

_____

_____

_____

_____

_____

Short-Term Objectives

_____

_____

_____

_____

_____

Long-Term Objectives

_____

_____

_____

_____

Planning

Step 3: What Services Will Achieve Your Goals?

Check off all the services that you either want to provide (column P) or that will achieve your goals (column G). You may find that you've checked off both boxes for each service. If you find that you have not checked off both boxes for a particular service, recognize the discrepancy.

P   G

☐ ☐ Newspaper editorials
☐ ☐ Group meetings
☐ ☐ House calls or visits/hospital visits
☐ ☐ Lectures/presentations
☐ ☐ Newsletter/publications
☐ ☐ Warmline
☐ ☐ Referrals
☐ ☐ Training
☐ ☐ Drop-in meetings
☐ ☐ Community groups
☐ ☐ Website
☐ ☐ Chat list
☐ ☐ Information on social networking sites
☐ ☐ Other _____

Postpartum Education for Parents

Postpartum Education for Parents (PEP) has been offering the following services since 1977: baby basics, new-parent groups, childbirth-class presentations, postpartum-distress support, and a free, 24-hour warmline service provides confidential, one-on-one support from trained volunteers who are parents.

Step 4: Compare and Contrast Organizations

List local resources that provide services similar to what you want your group to provide.

List the differences between those services and what your group proposes to provide. Use this information to: (1) get ideas from other established models and (2) avoid duplication of effort. Where does your group or network fit in?

This information can also be important in determining whether or not there are agencies who would like to sponsor or fund your endeavors. Your group may become a part of what those agencies offer. Depending on your committee's vision, assimilating into an existing agency may fulfill your goals. (For more on assimilation see Step 6B of Stage 3.)

Organization	Service Differences (Gaps in Service, What is Not Offered?)

Step 5: Seek Locations

Determine What's Available

To find a location, check with hospitals, birthing centers, churches and synagogues, local banks (they are often required to provide meeting rooms to charities), community mental health centers, libraries, schools, town halls, community colleges, and the YMCA/YWCA. Each location will have pros and cons. For example, a location may be near a bus line, have a large room, and is air conditioned. These would be pros. The cons may be limited parking, fee for room, no handicap access, or the room is available at odd hours only. List possible locations and their pros and cons below.

Organization _____

Address _____ Phone _____ Contact _____

Pros _____ Cons _____

Organization _____

Address _____ Phone _____ Contact _____

Pros _____ Cons _____

Social media can also help you find a place to meet. The Meetup.com website (*http://www.meetup.com*) helps groups gather every day in cafes, restaurants, and theaters for play dates, running meets, parties, workshops, conferences, and everything in between. In South Florida, a Postpartum Depression Network mom-to-mom support group was formed through *meetup.com/sfppdnetwork*.

Set Location, Day, and Time
When you decide on a location, propose days and times to your network. From there you can set the final days and times for your meetings.
List possible days and times for your meetings.

Possible Day	Times

Step 6. Beyond the Core Committee

Planning Your Group/Network Structure

You've investigated your ideas--now's the time to formalize the structure. You can continue to work as a separate entity, or assimilate into another organization. Either way, you need to create a permanent structure that will be maintained even when the charter members are no longer active in the group. This means working to cooperate as a whole, not as individuals. It's another step in recognizing and accomplishing your goals. You can operate as a charitable organization during start up, but in terms of long-term goals, it helps to know where you are headed.

A. Continuing as a Separate Group

Decide what your group's financial/tax status will be. Do you want the advantages and disadvantages of being a for-profit group or a non-profit/non-governmental organization (NGO)?

1. For-profit status

Investigate continuing your group as a company or corporation. You may need to consult business professionals, such as accountants and attorneys, about establishing a business. There are many websites designed to assist in this process.

List the advantages and disadvantages of becoming a for-profit group.

Advantages _____

_____

_____

Disadvantages _____

_____

_____

Is becoming a for-profit group consistent with the group's PPGO?

_____

_____

2. Non-profit Status

Governments oversee the tax status of nongovernment agencies (NGOs), charitable trusts, and non-profit oranizations. Investigate whether or not becoming a non-profit agency will serve your best interests. *http://citmedialaw.org/legal-guide/non-profit-legal-assistance* and *http://foundationcenter.org/getstarted/faqs/html/probono.html* are two helpful websites.

List the advantages and disadvantages of becoming a non-profit group.

Advantages	Disadvantages

Is becoming a non-profit group consistent with your group's purpose and philosophy?

_____

_____

Bylaws

Bylaws or a constitution are necessary for the governance and structure of a non-profit group. These will describe your organization's structure, officers, standing committees, and how initiatives are approved. Visit your local library or non-profit resource center for details on writing the rules that will govern your group or network. You might ask similar organizations for a copy of their bylaws as a template for developing your own.

Who in your group will be responsible for writing the bylaws?

_____

_____

By what date will the bylaws be completed?

_____

Which organizations can we contact for sample bylaws?

_____

_____

Governing Board of Directors or Trustees

Individuals must assume responsibility, both legally and ethically, for the group or network. The process of writing a constitution, or bylaws, will guide this important step.

According to your bylaws, how many directors do we need?

_____

_____

How often will they meet? Will meetings be in person or online?

_____

_____

_____

Who from the organizing committee has agreed to become part of your board?

_____

_____

_____

Who from outside the organizing committee has agreed to become part of your board?

_____

_____

_____

How will officers be selected?

_____

_____

_____

43

Decision-making

Will decisions be made by consensus, majority vote, or individuals? By an executive committee or by the organization as a whole? Will you hire staff or will volunteers run the group? Will there be different decision-making structures for different services?

What roles will volunteers play, if any?

_____

_____

_____

_____

_____

Will there be paid staff?

_____

_____

_____

_____

_____

What roles will paid staff play, if any?

_____

_____

_____

_____

_____

What roles will healthcare professionals play?

_____

_____

_____

_____

_____

B. Assimilation/Association with an Existing Group

Assimilation is a possibility if you don't want to be a separate group.

1. List the organizations, contact people, and decision-making bodies with which you could associate. Review the organizations you listed in Stage 3, Step 4.

Organization	Contact	Who Decides

2. List the pros and cons of becoming part of an existing agency/group.

Advantages could include expansion of services while saving money, increasing resources, broadening outreach; disadvantages might be loss of identity, reduced influence, needing to follow a different agenda.

Pros	Cons

Step 7: Formalize a Budget

It is essential that someone on your committee has experience with financial matters. Fiscal responsibility is a requirement for the whole group. Develop a budget for the first 12 months of operation.

Who in your group will develop the budget?

_____

_____

Possible Items for the Budget

Revenue	Expenses
Dues, fees	Staff salaries
Donations	Bank charges
Fundraising events	Fundraising events
Grants	Printing, brochures
Revenue from selling items	Postage
	Telephone/Internet service
	Training events
	Continuing education charges
	Rent and utilities
	Child-care worker
	Newsletter publication
	Office supplies
	Web design
	Website hosting
	Advertising
	Awards, thank-you gifts

Step 8: Open a Bank Account

The type of account you open for your group will depend on your tax status (i.e., for-profit or non-profit). Before you establish yourself as a non-profit organization, get a tax ID number to open a checking account. Different banks offer different services and values for personal, business, and non-profit accounts; investigate the banks in your own area.

Who in your group will be responsible for the account?

_____

_____

_____

Who will write checks and make withdrawals? Will checks require two signatures?

_____

_____

_____

_____

What kind of account will we have?

_____

_____

_____

_____

What will the banking fees be?

_____

_____

_____

_____

Will there be other restrictions on your account?

_____

_____

_____

_____

Step 9 Seek Funding

Develop fundraising strategies according to the stated budget. There are many options available to get income for your group, such as pooling money, holding fundraising events, and applying for grants.

Donations

Organizers or other interested individuals may contribute money as donations. It's not unusual for members of the Board of Directors or Trustees to make a written commitment to make sizable donations on a regular basis. Non-profit organizations enjoy tax-exempt status so they can receive these donations.

Events

There's practically no limit to fundraising events. Visit your library for books concerning fundraising, or hire a consultant. Read your local newspaper for ideas.

Grant Writing

A non-profit organization can obtain grants from local, state, and federal governments and from non-government foundations. Other sources of revenue are churches, service organizations, and clubs. Your local library will have resources on writing proposals for grants. Once you receive your first grant, you'll receive information from other grant sources automatically.

Caution

Grants can be time-consuming, difficult to obtain, and they often come with "strings attached." They are not a reliable income source for sustainability.

48

Membership

Requesting dues from current members of the group or network provides a steady source of income. The governing board determines the amount. There can be differing levels of membership dues depending upon members' ability to pay. For example, a non-wage-earner might pay less than a fully employed professional. In exchange for the dues payment, members receive products or services.

Postpartum Support International

Postpartum Support International (PSI) designates membership levels of student ($25), non-professional ($60), support group ($75), professional ($150), and for-profit ($250). The benefits of membership, available only to paying members, are a newsletter and discounts at the annual conference.

Step 10: Recruit Volunteers and/or Hire Staff

Recruit Volunteers

Volunteers may come from the general community or from your target population. They may be people who have received professional care in the past and are now fully functioning. They could work full time, part time, or not be currently employed. All will have obligations outside of your group. They will still have to meet the criteria of commitment and time, but are joining after the core committee has created the group or network.

Write the names and phone numbers of people already interested in volunteering.

Name	Phone	Email

Design Your Volunteer Application Process

It's important to formalize this process for practical as well as philosophical reasons. Develop a written application for all volunteers to complete. Keep in mind that you and the applicant are trying to find a match between the organization and the potential volunteer. The written application will inform both parties of expectations and level of commitment. See Appendix C for samples.

Check which topics will be addressed in your volunteer application.

YES or NO

- ☐ ☐ Times available/time commitment
- ☐ ☐ Types of service interested in providing
- ☐ ☐ Strengths: what the volunteer brings to the organization
- ☐ ☐ Weaknesses: what areas the volunteer can develop further
- ☐ ☐ Why is he or she interested in volunteering for this group?
- ☐ ☐ Other groups he or she has been involved in, and in what capacity
- ☐ ☐ Ethical standards
- ☐ ☐ Personal philosophy/values
- ☐ ☐ Personal background
- ☐ ☐ Personal references
- ☐ ☐ Professional background
- ☐ ☐ Leadership ability/commitment, if any
- ☐ ☐ Knowledge/background concerning the topic of the group
- ☐ ☐ Other current commitments

Who do you expect to volunteer?
Availability, background, values, or knowledge of topic.

_____

_____

Publicize Your Need for Volunteers

To recruit volunteers, follow the advice of Stage 1, Step 2 for finding others. Recognize that once the organization is established and providing services, it will be easier to recruit subsequent generations of volunteers.

What will you expect from your group's volunteers?

_____

_____

What role(s) will the group's volunteers play?

_____

_____

Will different volunteers have different roles?

_____

_____

What will the group offer volunteers?

_____

_____

Reviewing the Completed Applications

Who from your group will review the applications?

_____

_____

How will the completed applications be evaluated?

_____

_____

Conduct In-Person or Telephone Interviews

Make sure your group is clear about the obligations that it expects from each volunteer, and that your group is clear about what each volunteer expects in return. Even if such questions regarding time commitments, leadership commitments, and ethical standards seem like they were addressed in the written application, now is the time to reiterate your group's values and expectations of its volunteers and to ask more in-depth questions of the applicant.

Who from your group will call the applicants and set up interviews?

_____

_____

_____

Who will conduct the interviews?

_____

_____

_____

Will the interviews be conducted in person, or by telephone?

_____

_____

_____

Design a Written Volunteer Agreement to Be Signed

Develop a short written agreement that outlines your group's expectations of its volunteers. During the volunteer interview, discuss its points and ask the volunteer to sign the written agreement. See Appendix C for samples.

What expectations will be included in the written agreement?

_____
_____
_____

Staff Recruitment

The governing body determines job descriptions and salaries. A personnel committee may be established to oversee the process of recruitment and hiring. Recruiting appropriate candidates for position is a critical process. Legal advice may be required.

What positions does your group need filled by staff?

_____
_____
_____

Who will write the job descriptions?

_____
_____
_____

Who will be on the personnel committee?

_____
_____
_____

Has someone in the group obtained legal advice about recruitment?

_____
_____
_____

Step 11: Provide Training and Orientation to Volunteers/Staff

Share your knowledge and the group's purpose and goals. Decide whether or not your group's training procedure will:

1. Be designed by your group

2. Use existing community training

3. Be bought from outside organizations

Who from your group will contact community and outside resources for appropriate staff and volunteer training?

_____

_____

Will you design and use your own training, or use existing training from other community agencies?

_____

_____

Will you design and use your own training manual, or buy and use another group's training manual?

_____

_____

If you decide to create your own manual and provide your own training, who from your group will do that?

_____

_____

Will you have separate and/or different training for volunteers and staff?

_____

_____

> In 2012, Postpartum Education for Parents (PEP) launched the Baby Steps Project. The purpose is to inspire others to create a parent-support network, and customize it to fit another community. Their training curriculum, Developing Your Organization, has a CD with a complete set of documents in an electronic format for easy editing.

Volunteer Training

Check the topics that are important for your group to include in volunteer training.

YES or NO

☐ ☐ Expectations of the organization
☐ ☐ Times available/time commitment
☐ ☐ Referral techniques
☐ ☐ Expectations of the volunteers
☐ ☐ Local resources
☐ ☐ Active listening skills
☐ ☐ Confidentiality
☐ ☐ Group dynamics skills
☐ ☐ Recordkeeping
☐ ☐ Other: _____

Who will be in charge of the training?

_____

Will it be in person or online?

_____

Who will be the trainer?

_____

Is the trainer from inside or outside the group?

_____

When will the first training take place? (dates and times)

_____

Where will it take place?

_____

Will there be one or more meetings per training session?

_____

Will refreshments be provided?

_____

If so, who will provide them?

_____

What materials/handouts will the trainees receive?

_____

_____

Will certificates of completion be awarded?

_____

Costs for Volunteer Training

Trainer	$_____
Site Online Costs	+$_____
Handouts/Refreshments	+$_____
Other Materials	+$_____
Certificates	+$_____
Other Costs	+$_____
Total Training Costs	=$_____

Staff Training

Check the topics that are important for your group to include in staff training.

YES or NO

- ☐ ☐ Expectations of the organization
- ☐ ☐ Referral techniques
- ☐ ☐ Expectations of the staff
- ☐ ☐ Local resources
- ☐ ☐ Active listening skills
- ☐ ☐ Confidentiality
- ☐ ☐ Group dynamics skills
- ☐ ☐ Recordkeeping
- ☐ ☐ Office protocol
- ☐ ☐ Employee protocol
- ☐ ☐ Other: _____

Who will be in charge of the training?

_____

Who will be the trainer?

_____

Is the trainer from inside or outside the group?

_____

When will the first training take place? (dates and times)

_____

Where will it take place?

_____

Will there be one or more meetings per training session?

_____

What materials/handouts will the trainees receive?

_____

Costs for Staff Training

Trainer	$_____
Site Handouts	+$_____
Refreshments	+$_____
Other Materials	+$_____
Certificates	+$_____
Other Costs	+$_____
Total Training Costs	=$_____

STAGE 4.

Implementation

STEP 1:   Establish an Advisory Board of
           Supportive Community Professionals

STEP 2:   Create Printed or Online Materials

STEP 3:   Begin Publicity and Outreach to
           Target Population

STEP 4:   Initiate Operation and Service

Step 1: Establish an Advisory Board of Supportive Community Professionals

An advisory board is a group of professionals who have agreed to provide expertise when asked. The responsibilities of an advisory board are not to operate the group or network, but to provide support in times of regular operation and crisis, and to provide endorsements for your group. Such a board also provides credibility when fundraising. At this point in your process, you have gotten to know some of the interested or influential professionals in your area. Contact them about becoming a part of your advisory board. You don't need to limit your search to local experts. National or international experts can also be contacted and are often quite willing to help.

Professionals Willing to Become Members of our Advisory Board

Name	Organization (if any)	Phone Number	Email

How often will the advisory board meet, if at all?

_____

_____

Will the meeting be online or in person?

_____

_____

Who will lead the meetings?

_____

_____

Who determines the structure of the meetings?

_____

_____

Who will communicate with the advisory board? What types of communication will they receive? How often?

_____

_____

_____

Will there be a listserv for advisory board members?

_____

Step 2: Create Printed or Online Materials

Not only will your group or network want to provide emotional support to the beneficiaries of your group, they'll want to give information as well. Printed or online materials are an effective way to educate parents and your community.

Types of Information to Provide

There are four types of information that your organization may want to disseminate:

1. The topic
2. Your organization
3. Ways to contribute
4. Resources and referrals

1. Topic

If your organization's focus is on postpartum depression or anxiety, the literature you produce could include a description of postpartum depression and anxiety, methods of treatment, coping strategies, and self-screening tools. You might develop several free handouts and have them available on your website.

2. Resources and Referrals

Resources and referrals can include a list of phone numbers and websites that parents can use in times of need (local hospital, helpline, warmline), and a list of referral agencies or professionals.

3. Your Group/Network

Your organizational literature (in print or online) should include information about your group, such as your organization's name, fees or dues, days and times of operation, location, purpose or philosophy, and the services you provide.

4. Ways to Contribute

This information will guide prospective volunteers and individuals in how to volunteer or make financial donations. This is invaluable for a group that works solely from membership dues.

Describe the type(s) of information you want to have available in print or online formats.

- Topic _____
  Definitions, coping strategies

  _____

  _____

- Resources/referrals _____
  Other groups, phone numbers, books

  _____

  _____

- Your group/network _____
  Group name, phone number, purpose

  _____

  _____

- Ways to contribute _____
  Ways to donate money, volunteer time

  _____

  _____

How will it be distributed?

_____

_____

_____

Who will receive your materials? Check all that apply.

- ☐ Beneficiaries of service
- ☐ Potential volunteers
- ☐ Healthcare professionals
- ☐ Potential donors
- ☐ Referral sources
- ☐ Visitors to your website

- ☐ Other _____

How and when will they receive your materials ? Check all that apply.

- ☐ Lectures/presentations put on by your group
- ☐ Lectures/presentations put on by other groups
- ☐ During services provided by your group
- ☐ Hospital/home visits
- ☐ Support group meetings
- ☐ In a "welcome" package from the hospital after giving birth
- ☐ Downloads from your website
- ☐ Email
- ☐ During services provided from other groups or agencies
- ☐ One-on-one
- ☐ In a group
- ☐ By mail
- ☐ If by mail, who will pay for postage? _____
- ☐ Other _____

Who from your group will distribute the material?

_____

In New York, state legislators passed the Maternity Information Law that requires that all hospital and birth centers in New York State distribute to each prospective mother at the time of pre-registration a leaflet with definitions of maternity-related procedures and practices. It also includes a short description of PPD, and each facility can imprint its own group or agency information.

Format of Publications

Now that you've decided what type(s) of information to offer in print or online, consider what format will best communicate your message and reach your audience. Below are several types of publications and examples of how some organizations have used them.

Articles

The National Association of Mothers' Centers offers articles with useful information for mothers and parents collected from a variety of experts who have spoken at their seminars and conferences. You can find examples on their website: *http://.namc.org*

Blogs

Blogs provide an opportunity to reach a broad audience. If you have someone in your group who wants to regularly post on your blog, you might consider starting one. Really consider whether you have someone to keep up your blog. Many are started with good intentions and quickly die out, which does not reflect well on the organization.

Brochures and Printed Materials

Websites have, in many respects, replaced the printed brochure. However, you may still find that some printed materials are necessary. For example, you may wish to develop rack cards, postcards, or business cards with your organization name, contact information, and website address. These can be given directly to new families, professionals, or community members. Online printers, such as VistaPrint or 48-Hours, can produce your printed materials for relatively low cost.

Booklets, Books

Community bookstores, libraries, and online bookstores offer an increasing array of written materials for family support. For 55 years, *The Womanly Art of Breastfeeding*, 8th Edition, has provided support for breastfeeding mothers. It is available at *http://www.LLLI.org*.

Your organization might also consider having an Amazon affiliate bookstore on your website. This will allow you to sell books you recommend on your website and make a small profit. Amazon handles all order fulfillment. More information is available on the Amazon site. *https://affiliate-program.amazon.com/gp/associates/join/faq.html*

Newsletters

Newsletters can be another way to communicate with volunteers, donors, and families. They can be in print or electronic, and can be distributed monthly, bimonthly, or quarterly. Back issues can be posted on your organization's website.

> Postpartum Education for Parents' *News Notes* is emailed to current volunteers in Santa Barbara, California at the start of each month. It includes the warmline shift schedule, information about upcoming and past services and special events, recognition of individual volunteer efforts, and appeals for upcoming volunteer opportunities.
>
> Program for Early Parent Support has a quarterly newsletter that is an ongoing extension of PEPS resources, providing timely parenting information for families with kids of all ages, upcoming parenting lectures and events, plus access to a wealth of community resources. It is available on their website: *http://www.peps.org*

How will you create your printed materials or website content?

☐ Buy it from another organization?
☐ Link to an existing website?
☐ Write and design it yourselves?
☐ Pay someone to write and design it?

☐ Other? _____

Who will be in charge of developing and maintaining printed or online materials?

Printed Material

Who will write the content for printed material?

_____

_____

How much will it cost to design?

_____

_____

How much will it cost to print?

_____

_____

Who will distribute it?

_____

_____

How much will it cost to distribute?

_____

_____

Online Content

Who will design the website?

_____

_____

Who will maintain the website?

_____

_____

How much will it cost to design and maintain?

_____

_____

_____

Who will create and maintain your social media pages (Facebook, LinkedIn, Twitter)?

_____

_____

_____

Step 3: Begin Publicity and Outreach to Target Population

Publicity can consist of the same things that were suggested to recruit organizers (Stage 1) and volunteers (Stage 3). Paid advertisements can be placed in local newspapers. You can also get more elaborate by using fundraising events that local newspapers, radio, and television stations can publicize. You can use social media. Add content to your Facebook and Twitter pages on a regular basis to direct people to your website.

Other Ways to Spread the Word

Contacts in Your Workbook or Online Desktop

Look at the list of people in the file that you have kept from the beginning. Who are they? If you've completed the previous steps in this workbook, you already know some of the personnel at hospitals, doctors' offices, prenatal classes, social service agencies, and birthing centers to whom you can give your flyers, brochures, and other printed materials. Could they help you with public relations? Who do they know and what other contacts can they give you?

Places you have dropped off your flyer/brochure.

_____

_____

_____

_____

Organizations that will let us distribute or display your materials, publicize, link to your website (to increase visibility on search engines), ask people to publicize your group on social media.

_____

_____

_____

_____

_____

_____

> **Postpartum Education for Parents** (PEP) organizers in California have been able to get their information included in hospital "welcome" packages for new parents. In addition, they bought plastic containers to display their brochures and placed them in every obstetrician/gynecologist and pediatrician office in their community.

Presentations

Identify opportunities to give a talk about your group to service organizations, professional groups, religious institutions, and local clubs that meet regularly. Presentations can be local, national, or international. These events can raise awareness and may even aid in fundraising.

List organizations where someone from your group can make a presentation.

_____

_____

_____

_____

_____

_____

Public-Service Announcements (PSA) or Press Releases

Make it short and to the point. If you're unsure about what format to use, contact the advertising department of a television station or newspaper for instructions. Companies, such as PR Web, offer low-cost press releases that go to a wide range of media outlets. It is important to include the following information in your PSA or press release.

- Group name
- Location
- Dates and times of meetings
- Service(s) provided
- Contact information

Your community's media outlets and contact people.

Name	Medium	Company	Phone

Social Media

Do you have a Facebook page for your organization? A Twitter and LinkedIn Account?

_____

_____

_____

Who will post announcements for you?

_____

_____

_____

Step 4: Initiate Operation and Service

This is what you've been working toward. Organizers need to be patient during the beginning phase of operations. Ongoing projects can be helpful in this regard.

How can you keep morale up during the first months if there is low attendance or participation?

_____

_____

_____

_____

What projects do you have in the works?

_____

_____

_____

_____

What are you doing well?

_____

_____

_____

_____

What changes do you need to make?

_____

_____

_____

_____

Only two mothers attended the first Postpartum Education for Parents (PEP) support group when it was started in 1977. Although turnout was low in the beginning, PEP has served tens of thousands of families through its new-parent support groups in the Santa Barbara, California area.

STAGE 5.
Evaluation

STEP 1:   Design or Seek Evaluation Processes

STEP 2:   Outline Your Evaluation Process

STEP 3:   Consider Your Results

Step 1: Design or Seek Evaluation Processes

How Are You Doing? What Works? What Doesn't?

It's important that you find or create a system that will measure the successes and shortcomings of your group. You can get feedback for the evaluation process through internal and external sources. The results of your group or network's evaluations can strengthen the services, and evaluations are required if you are receiving money from an outside source. Don't try to avoid or casually neglect this step; it's vital to the future success of your group or network. It matters what others think about how your group has or hasn't assisted them.

Sources of Feedback
- Internal evaluations done by people within the organization
- External evaluations done by people outside the organization
- Telephone surveys
- Written or online questionnaires
- Your organization's Facebook page or Yelp profile
- Feedback from participants, organizers, and/or volunteers/survey/focus groups for non-participants
- Personnel reviews performed by a supervisor and/or members of a personnel committee appointed by the Board of Directors

Examples of External Evaluations
- Feedback from people who can refer your services to potential beneficiaries
- Feedback from healthcare and mental health professionals/ paraprofessionals
- Feedback from stakeholders

Evaluation Results You Need to Share with Your Funder

If you've received a grant to start your organization or provide services for your community, the organization you received the grant from may also require an evaluation of your program. Review those requirements from the grant-providing organization.

What type of feedback do you need to provide to your funder?

_____

_____

_____

_____

What You Can Learn from Other Organizations.

While networking, you may have spoken with individuals who would be willing and able to share their evaluation processes or forms. If necessary, they can refer you to an outside consultant.

Who is or may be willing to share their evaluation process/forms with your group?

Name	Organization	Phone	Email

What kind of evaluation processes do their groups use?

_____

_____

_____

What areas do they assess (services, staff, volunteers, etc.)?

_____

_____

_____

Step 2: Outline Your Evaluation Process

Will you do an internal or external evaluation?

_____

Who will administer the evaluation process?

Your evaluation process will encourage recommendations for which of the following? Check all that apply.

☐
☐ Needs assessment
☐ Accessibility of services
☐ Existing services
☐ Future services

Other: _____

Check the area(s) of your group or network that will be evaluated.

☐
☐ Staff
☐ Organizational structure
☐ Volunteers
☐ Training process
☐ Accessibility of services
☐ Current provision of services

☐ Other: _____

Other: _____

Feedback from your evaluation will be sent to:

☐
☐ Stakeholders
☐ Participants
☐ Outside consultants
☐ Organizers
☐ Your advisory board
☐ Volunteers
☐ Funders

☐ Other: _____

Other: _____

Step 3: Consider Your Results

What did you learn from the evaluation?

_____

_____

_____

_____

_____

What changes might occur as a result?

_____

_____

_____

_____

_____

_____

STAGE 6.
Future Endeavors

STEP 1:   Develop Partnerships

STEP 2:   Establish New Goals and Objectives

STEP 3:   Write Your own Manual on How You
           Started Your Group

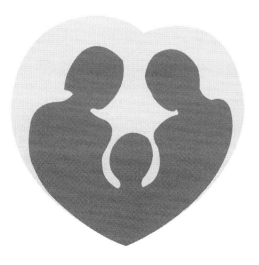

Step 1: Develop Partnerships

Taking the partnership or team approach means superior service for the target population. Explore whether other organizations in your community would be interested in becoming partners. Develop partnerships between your group or network and healthcare professionals. These should benefit both groups. Ideally, you'll want to partner with groups whose services overlap with yours.

What do you hope to achieve by collaborating?

_____

_____

_____

_____

_____

With what organizations would you like your group to collaborate? Assess how connected you have become through this development process.

_____

_____

_____

_____

_____

Would you like to collaborate with another group on a project? What type of project?

_____

_____

_____

_____

_____

Who are the key people (in your group and outside it) making such projects and collaborations happen?

_____

_____

_____

_____

Step 2: Establish New Goals and Objectives

Once your group is well established and has been evaluated, you may want to formulate new goals and objectives. Those that you created in the beginning helped you to start the group, but a change in your focus may occur in the future to reflect a new or modified vision of how to continue the group. Events out of your control can affect outcomes, so be flexible!

Postpartum Health Alliance of California was originally founded to address the needs of parents in the Sacramento Valley, but quickly spread to the rest of Northern California and eventually, grew to serve all of California. PHA's original goals when the group started in 1994 were to:

1. Improve availability, accessibility, distribution of information, and resources
2. Improve coordination between professionals, consumers, and available resources
3. Increase incidence of early identification, intervention, and referrals

In 1998, PHA developed new goals and objectives for 1999. They included a project to launch warmlines in the San Francisco Bay and Los Angeles areas, form board committees, increase membership, and solicit funds/grant writing. They redefined their purpose and have reviewed their mission statement.

Has your original vision changed? How?

_____

_____

_____

What are some possible new directions for your organization?

_____

_____

_____

_____

79

Are there new projects you would like your group to undertake?

_____

_____

_____

_____

Does your mission statement reflect your new priorities and goals?

_____

_____

_____

_____

Step 3: Write Your Own Manual on How You Started Your Group

Your experience in reaching this final step is unique. You have achieved your goal. Congratulations! Your group or network's history may be helpful to others, so consider putting your accumulated knowledge into a format that others can access and use. Knowledge is power. You are now in a position to empower others.

Who will write your manual of how you established your organization?

_____

_____

How will you disseminate it to others?

_____

_____

_____

_____

Thank you for your contribution to the support of families around the world.

STAGE A.

Committee Activity

Your Experiences, Skills, and Proficiencies

Read through the table. This list will help you match your skills with the tasks that need to be done. Rate yourself for each skill or experience. Feel free to add other skills at the bottom of the list. When you're finished, circle your strengths, then highlight which skills need improvement. When it comes time to volunteer for tasks, choose those that not only match your strengths, but that will provide opportunities for growth.

Personal Experiences and Characteristics

Please rate each as experience or characteristic as ranging from "Not True for Me" to "Very True for Me" on a 5-point scale.

(1=Not True for Me, 5 = Very True for Me)

Enthusiasm/passion for parenting

1	2	3	4	5
Not True for Me			*Very True for Me*	

Willingness to learn

1	2	3	4	5

Experience in creating a support group

1	2	3	4	5

Like to talk

1	2	3	4	5

People skills

1	2	3	4	5

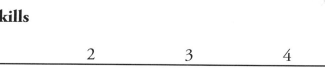

Know a lot of people

1   2   3   4   5
Not True for Me   *Very True for Me*

Comfortable with strangers

1   2   3   4   5

Commitment to taking care of others

1   2   3   4   5

Commitment to taking care of myself

1   2   3   4   5

Survivor of pregnancy and/or postpartum depression or anxiety

1   2   3   4   5

Experienced breastfeeding difficulties

1   2   3   4   5

Abuse survivor

1   2   3   4   5

Helped someone with breastfeeding difficulties

1   2   3   4   5

Helped someone with pre and/or postpartum depression/anxiety

1   2   3   4   5

Organizational Skills

Please rate each skill below as ranging from "Not Skilled" to "Very Skilled" on a 5-point scale.

(1 = Not Skilled, 5 = Very Skilled)

Financial expertise

1	2	3	4	5
Not Skilled				*Very Skilled*

Event planning

1	2	3	4	5

Conference organizing

1	2	3	4	5

Computer skills

1	2	3	4	5

Public speaking

1	2	3	4	5

Leadership skills

1	2	3	4	5

Fundraising skills

1	2	3	4	5

Web design

1	2	3	4	5

Graphic design

1	2	3	4	5

Not Skilled   *Very Skilled*

Accounting software

1	2	3	4	5

Legal skills

1	2	3	4	5

PowerPoint

1	2	3	4	5

Short-term planning skills and focus

1	2	3	4	5

Long-term planning skills and focus

1	2	3	4	5

Knowledge of mental health issues

1	2	3	4	5

Once this list is completed, make a list of your strengths to help you find the right volunteer opportunities.

STAGE B.

List of Organizations

DONA International
35 E. Wacker Dr., Ste. 850
Chicago, IL 60601-2106

(888) 788-DONA (3662)
Fax: (312) 644-8557
Web: *www.dona.org*

La Leche League International
957 N. Plum Grove Road
Schaumburg, IL 60173

(847) 519-7730 or (800) LALECHE (*525-3243*)
Fax: (847) 969-0460
Customer service: (847) 519-9585
Web: *www.llli.org*

Lamaze International
2025 M Street NW Suite 800
Washington, DC 20036-3309

Toll free: (800) 368-4404
Phone: (202) 367-1128
Fax: (202) 367-2128
Web: *www.lamazeinternational.org*

Motherwoman
Mailing Address
P.O. Box 2635
Amherst, MA 01004

Office Adddress
220 Russell St. (Rt. 9), Suite 200
Hadley, MA, 01035

Phone: (413) 387-0703 Fax: (413) 306-3175
Email: *info@motherwoman.org* Web: *www.motherwoman.org*

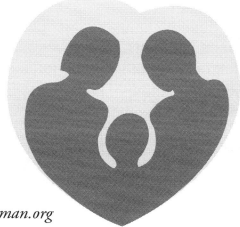

National Association of Mothers' Centers (NAMC)
1740 Old Jericho Turnpike
Jericho, NY 11753

(877) 939-MOMS
(516) 750-5365 (fax)
www.motherscenters.org

Pacific Postpartum Support Society (PPPSS)
7342 Winston Street, Suite 200
Burnaby, BC V5A 2H1
CANADA

Business line: (604) 255-7955
Fax: (604) 255-7588
Email: *admin@postpartum.org*

Postpartum Education for Parents (PEP)
PO Box 261
Santa Barbara, CA 93116

PEP Warmline: (805) 564-3888
Email: *pepboard@sbpep.org* Web: *www.sbpep.org*

Postpartum Support International (PSI)
6706 SW 54th Avenue
Portland, Oregon 97219

PSI Office Telephone: (503) 894-9453
Fax: (503) 894-9452
Support Helpline: (800) 944-4PPD *(4773)*
Web: *www.postpartum.net*

Program for Early Parent Support
4649 Sunnyside Avenue North, # 324
Seattle, WA 98103-6900

Telephone: (206) 547-8570
Snohomish County Line: (425) 744-1199
Fax: (206) 633-2179
Email: *PEPS@peps.org* Web: *www.peps.org*

STAGE C.
Volunteer Forms

Sample Volunteer Application
Source: Postpartum Education for Parents

Name _____ Spouse _____

Address _____ Phone _____

Age and sex of children _____

We are happy that you are interested in becoming a volunteer. We think it is important for our volunteers to examine and understand how they feel about their own parenthood experiences and their motives for volunteering before they begin talking to other parents. We would like you to answer the following questions. We will discuss them further when we meet you before training begins. If necessary, use the back of this form to complete your answers.

Why do you want to be a volunteer?

_____

_____

What do you think you can contribute? What are some of your strengths and weaknesses?

_____

_____

What do you expect to gain from being a volunteer?

_____

_____

Briefly describe your feelings as a new parent.

_____

_____

What have you learned from being a parent? How and why has it helped you grow?

_____

_____

What is the best approach to parenting? What do new parents most need to know?

_____

_____

Are you willing to make a commitment as a volunteer for one year?

_____

_____

Please return this application by _____

to: _____

Sample Volunteer Commitment Sheet

The following services are offered free of charge to all interested parents in the community.
- Telephone Support
- New-Parent Discussion Groups
- Speaker for Childbirth-Preparation Class
- Special Circumstances Facilitators
- Home Support

Volunteers are recruited, screened, interviewed, and trained to provide the above services. All volunteers are expected to do telephone duty. Volunteers may also perform other duties in the organization's administration, or other services depending on interest and training.

Volunteers are asked to make the following commitment
One year of service, including:
- Initial training
- No more than six telephone shifts per month
- No more than one in-service training meeting per month

When on duty, volunteers will:
Call in to the Volunteer Coordinator (or answering service, if used).
> Volunteers may leave their posts as necessary during the shift, but must notify the Volunteer Coordinator or answering service of the expected length of absence, or leave a number where he or she can be reached. Upon returning, volunteers should report back in.

STRICT CONFIDENTIALITY IS ADHERED TO AT ALL TIME.

We do not endorse or recommend doctors, psychologists or counselors, nurses, hospitals, dentists, lawyers, or other professionals or agencies.

Sample Volunteer Acceptance Letter

[date]

Dear Volunteer:

Congratulations! We are pleased to welcome you to the growing number of volunteers at [name of organization].

A training workshop has been scheduled for [date, time, place].

A reading unit and other background materials are included with [this letter or attached to an email]. Please read them before attending the workshop.

Please bring a sandwich to contribute to a sandwich tray for lunch. We will provide fruit, beverages, and other refreshments.

Training is an event that all our volunteers thoroughly enjoy, and we are looking forward to sharing it with you.

Sincerely,

[signature]
Volunteer Coordinator

Also from Praeclarus Press

The Virtual Breastfeeding Culture
Seeking Mother-to-Mother Support in the Digital Age

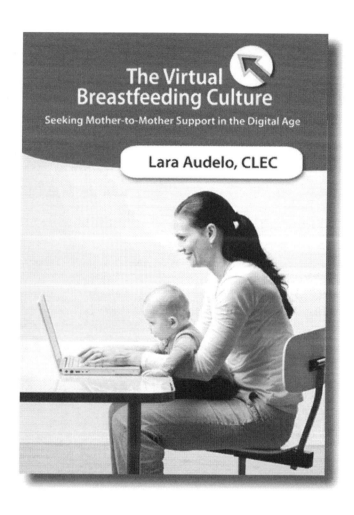

The Virtual Breastfeeding Culture: Seeking Mother-to-Mother Support in the Digital Age illustrates that since the advent of the digital communication, mothers have been using the Internet to support and connect with each other. Women have claimed the Internet as their own, and have created an elaborate infrastructure of virtual support.

Virtual Breastfeeding Culture *is a clarion call to change the way we support expecting and new mothers, and is a valuable addition to the breastfeeding-support library.*

—Danielle Rigg, JD, CLC and Bettina Forbes, CLC, Best for Babes Foundation

To order a copy visit our at www.praeclaruspress.com website or for a complete list of our books visit our website by scanning the QR code below.

Praeclarus Press publishes books that change people's lives. We want our books to be engaging, grabbing the reader's attention, and beautiful, to nourish their spirits. Smart, but still accessible and practical. Compassionate, while reflecting a solid base in evidence. In short, we want them to be excellent.

All of our books are also available
for order at www.amazon.com